ASHLEY BARANDIARAN

A Beginner's Handbook to Non-Toxic Living

Making the Switch to Natural Home, Body, and Wellness Products

Copyright © 2024 by Ashley Barandiaran

All rights reserved. No part of this publication may be reproduced, stored or transmitted in any form or by any means, electronic, mechanical, photocopying, recording, scanning, or otherwise without written permission from the publisher. It is illegal to copy this book, post it to a website, or distribute it by any other means without permission.

First edition

This book was professionally typeset on Reedsy. Find out more at reedsy.com

Contents

Preface	v
Prologue	1
Introduction	3
1 Understanding Our Exposures	4
1.1 Navigating a Toxic World	4
1.2 Commonly Used Irritants Explained	5
2 Crafting your Non-toxic Living Space: Transitioning to a...	8
2.1 Purifying your Living Space	8
2.2 Detoxifying Your Bedroom for Better Sleep	14
2.3 The Kitchen Haul: Swapping for Safer Cookware, Utensils, and Cleaners	16
2.4 Decoding Food: Having Healthier Eating Habits	18
3 Non-Toxic Cleaning & Laundry: A Healthier Choice for You and...	27
4 Nurturing Your Body: Understanding The Good, The Bad, and...	33
4.1 Natural Skin, Hair, and Dental Care Solutions	33
4.2 Personal Care Essentials: Beauty Products: Skincare & Cosmetics	37
4.3 Homemade Beauty: Simple Recipes for Skincare	38
4.4 Good Clothing Habits & Upcycling Clothing	40
4.5 Natural First Aid and Holistic Remedies	41
5 Prioritizing Wellness	45
5.1 Free Natural Shifts	46

5.2 Dr. Ashley's Personal Favorites 47
6 Conclusion 51
References 54

Preface

Welcome to The Beginner's Guide to Non-Toxic Living. My name is Dr. Ashley Barandiaran and I am very excited about writing this book. For one, now I have a pocketbook guide I can share with family, friends, and patients on ways to live a healthier and more sustainable life and move towards a lifestyle minimizing toxins benefiting their health and the Earth. And two, I can share this information with a larger audience driven to create a healthier, safer world for themselves and future generations.

Brief background

I am a dedicated Doctor of Chinese Medicine and Acupuncturist in San Diego. My journey into alternative health began early, driven by my younger sibling's severe illness as an infant. When Western medicine reached its limits, my family turned to alternative treatments, which resulted in my sister surpassing her developmental milestones and becoming seizure-free. As a family, we continued alternative medicine to support our health journeys. This is what inspired my lifelong commitment to alternative medicine

My personal health journey took a significant turn when I was involved in a car accident and sustained a neck injury. From personal experience, I witnessed firsthand the quality of care acupuncture offers and its ability to integrate both Eastern and Western medicine. I believe it provides unparalleled care treating all aspects required for healing: body, mind, and spirit.

I love being a practitioner in this field because it is a preventative health modality that works to treat current medical needs naturally, safely, and effectively. I love empowering my patients and acting as a conduit for their healing journey. I find it so rewarding to provide quality care by integrating Western science with Traditional Chinese Medicine, adapting a 3000-year-old medicine to current medical needs.

Outside of my practice, I enjoy connection with my community, home-cooked meals, an active outdoor lifestyle, travel, yoga, Pilates, live music, and dancing. Deeply rooted in my hometown, I cherish community involvement and volunteer work. I am passionate about giving back to my community. This passion for sustainability and minimizing toxins has grown throughout the years and this is something I would like to share.

This journey has not only led me to take care of my body but it has also opened doors to caring for our Earth even more and supporting like-minded products & people. My goal with this is to introduce lasting practices and products that are beneficial long-term to our health and world. I want to make this an easy transition, making lasting changes in the home, where we have control and spend most of our time.

Prologue

In this book, you'll find at the foundation, a real-life experience; both first-hand and that of my community. Through this, I will be sharing with you personal solutions, insights, and real health data you won't find just by searching the web

Structured to be your companion rather than a textbook, each chapter of this book builds on the last, gradually equipping you with the knowledge and confidence to make healthier choices. Whether you're looking to overhaul your cleaning cabinet or find natural skincare options that work, you'll find actionable steps to take you there. And remember, it's all about baby steps. You don't have to do it all at once.

I encourage you, as you turn these pages, to start with one small change. Maybe it's swapping out your empty detergent with a clean biodegradable one or trying to make your very own sunscreen. Whatever it is, celebrate that step, because it's a step toward a healthier you and a healthier world.

I'm also extending an invitation to join our online community, where you can share your triumphs, swap tips, and find encouragement on those days when it all seems a bit daunting. Together, we can make a difference, not just in our homes but in the world. Throughout this book, I will make recommendations to help you navigate your journey toward a healthier, non-toxic lifestyle.

To make this even easier, I've included a QR code that links to a curated selection of products I love, these are items I use and recommend. These products align with the principles of holistic health and environmental sustainability that I advocate. Simply scan the QR code to explore and purchase items that will support your transition to a non-toxic lifestyle.

Are you ready to take the first step toward a healthier, safer world? Let's dive in together and create positive change, one small adjustment at a time.

  -Dr. Ashley Barandiaran

Introduction

Welcome to your journey toward a non-toxic lifestyle! In this book, we'll explore how to transition to a healthier, safer home environment—starting with the place where we have the most control. Remember, the goal is progress, not perfection. Make changes that resonate with you, and consider replacing items one at a time as you start running low. This approach keeps the process manageable and enjoyable.

By making conscious choices about the products we use and the materials we surround ourselves with, we can significantly reduce our exposure to harmful chemicals and improve our overall health and well-being.

Getting Started:

My best advice is to start in your home. As you run out of a product, begin replacing it with natural, non-toxic alternatives. Beginners often buy products labeled "green" or "natural" without fully understanding what they're purchasing, leading to skepticism and disappointment. This book aims to provide vetted resources and knowledge so you can make informed decisions for years to come.

Let's embark on this journey together and create a healthier, happier home!

1

Understanding Our Exposures

1.1 Navigating a Toxic World

Living in a world filled with toxins can have detrimental effects on our health. From the chemicals found in our cleaning supplies to those lurking in our personal care products, it's essential to understand the impact these substances can have on our well-being. Every day, we are exposed to chemicals that can potentially have harmful long-term effects. According to the Environmental Protection Agency, of the more than 40,000 chemicals used in consumer products in the US, less than 1% have been rigorously tested for human safety.

Did you know the average household contains about 62 toxic chemicals? These substances can significantly impact our health. Research shows that many of these compounds are irritants and carcinogens, capable of causing long-term health issues such as allergies, asthma, autoimmune disorders, organ damage, reproductive problems, and affecting the mental, intellectual, and physical development of children.

Understanding and reducing our exposure to these toxins is essential for maintaining a healthy home environment. This book aims to guide you through practical steps and simple swaps to minimize the presence of harmful chemicals in your home, ultimately enhancing your family's well-being.

One significant group of harmful compounds that often goes unnoticed is endocrine disruptors. These chemicals interfere with the body's endocrine system, which regulates hormone production and function. Endocrine disruptors can mimic hormones in the body, leading to hormonal imbalances and a range of health issues. Common endocrine disruptors include pesticides, bisphenol-A (BPA), per- and polyfluoroalkyl substances (PFAS), phthalates, parabens, and flame retardants. These substances are part of our everyday environment and can significantly affect our health.

By understanding the risks and learning how to make informed choices, we can create a safer, healthier living space for ourselves and our loved ones. This book is here to help you navigate this journey with practical advice and simple changes that can make a big difference. Let's take the first step towards a toxin-free lifestyle together.

1.2 Commonly Used Irritants Explained

Understanding the toxins in our environment is essential for making informed choices about our health. Here's a friendly and informative guide to some commonly used chemical toxins:

BPA (Bisphenol A): BPA is found in food and beverage packaging, medical devices, thermal paper, and dental materials. It can contaminate food, drinks, air, and soil, accumulating in human tissues and organs. BPA mimics estrogen, binding to estrogen receptors and potentially influencing body weight and tumor formation.

PFAS (Per- and Polyfluoroalkyl Substances): Known as "forever chemicals," PFAS includes over 9,000 chemicals used to make products water, grease, stain, and heat resistant. Found in items like carpets, fabrics, cleaning products, and firefighting foams, PFAS are persistent in the environment. Almost all Americans have PFAS in their blood. Even low exposure over time can affect reproductive organs, kidneys, liver, hormones, birth outcomes, and immune function.

Flame Retardants: These chemicals are applied to materials to prevent or slow fire growth. They are used in furniture, mattresses, electronics, building materials, and clothing often made with formaldehyde, polyurethane foams, adhesives, and toxic fragrances. Synthetic materials with flame retardants can off-gas over time. Since 2007, mattresses must contain flame retardants to meet safety standards, but there's no regulation on the chemicals used.

Parabens: Parabens are artificial preservatives found in pharmaceuticals, cosmetics, body care products, and food. They can interfere with hormone function and production. Common types include methyl-, ethyl-, propyl-, isopropyl-, butyl-, and isobutylparaben.

Phthalates: These chemicals make plastic more durable and are found in cosmetics, food, pharmaceuticals, electronics, air fresheners, toys, and containers. Both parabens and phthalates are linked to cancer, reproductive complications, endocrine system disruptions, allergies, and respiratory problems. Phthalates are also connected to ADHD, obesity, type II diabetes, neurodevelopmental disorders, behavioral problems, and autism spectrum disorders.

Pesticides: Pesticides are used to eliminate, reduce, or repel pests. Their impact on health varies; organophosphates and carbamates can disrupt the nervous system, while others may cause skin or eye irritation. Some pesticides are carcinogenic, and others interfere with the endocrine system.

Environmental Exposure: We encounter chemical, biological, or physical elements in the air, water, food, or soil that can affect our health. This includes pesticides, personal care products with phthalates and parabens, plastics, flame retardants, BPA, and PFAS. Most of us are exposed to hundreds or thousands of these substances daily.

By understanding these toxins, we can take steps to minimize our exposure and protect our health.

2

Crafting your Non-toxic Living Space: Transitioning to a Non-Toxic Home Environment

Your home is your sanctuary, where you spend the majority of your time. It's crucial to ensure that it's a safe and healthy space for you and your loved ones. In this chapter, we'll dive into the different areas of your home where toxins can lurk, and we'll explore practical steps to minimize your exposure to harmful substances. I understand that you lead a busy life, striving for balance and intentionality while juggling multiple responsibilities. By making simple changes in your home environment, you can significantly improve your overall well-being. Let's simplify the process of creating a healthier home environment.

2.1 Purifying your Living Space

Ventilating

Ventilating is a simple yet effective way to minimize the toxin load in your home. Off-gassing refers to the process of allowing chemicals from common household items that emit strong odors to air out. By allowing these items to air out for hours to days, you can significantly reduce the presence of volatile organic compounds (VOCs) in the air.

Many daily use items such as paint, building materials, varnish, cleaning products, hairspray, and cosmetics contain harmful chemicals that can affect our health in the long term. To minimize VOCs in your home, consider the following steps:

1. <u>Airing Out Furniture</u>: Before bringing new furniture into your home, allow it to air out in a well-ventilated area. Opt for furniture made from natural sources like genuine leather or solid wood, and check labels for indications such as "contains no added flame retardants."
2. <u>Increasing Ventilation</u>: Keep windows open to facilitate airflow and allow fresh air to vent outdoors. This helps to dilute indoor air pollutants and maintain a healthier indoor environment.
3. <u>Adopting a Minimal Lifestyle</u>: Having fewer possessions not only reduces clutter but also minimizes the number of items off-gassing harmful chemicals in your home.
4. <u>Regular Cleaning Practices</u>: Mopping, washing your hands frequently, and using a vacuum equipped with a HEPA filter can help to remove dust and airborne particles, reducing the concentration of fumes in the air.

By implementing these simple strategies, you can take proactive steps to reduce off-gassing in your home and create a healthier living environment for you and your family.

Removing shoes

Removing shoes before entering your home is one of the simplest yet most effective steps you can take to create a cleaner and healthier living environment. By leaving your shoes at the door, you're not only reducing the amount of time spent cleaning, but you're also preventing the entry of thousands of germs, toxins, viruses, dust, dirt, and pesticides from the outside world.

Designating indoor slippers for yourself adds an extra layer of comfort and cleanliness. Consider setting up a shoe station near the main entryway with a basket of washable knit slippers in various sizes for guests to use. For optimal foot care, opt for wool or organic cotton socks. While it may be challenging to find non-toxic shoes, you can limit off-gassing in your home by storing shoes in the garage or a designated bin. Additionally, maintaining a minimal shoe selection helps minimize the introduction of chemicals and dirt into your living space.

Minimizing electromagnetic field (EMF) exposure:

In today's tech-driven world, we're constantly surrounded by electromagnetic fields (EMFs) from our gadgets, Wi-Fi routers, and powerlines. While these advancements make our lives easier, there are growing concerns about their impact on our health. Even though EMFs are invisible, they're everywhere, interacting with our bodies in ways we're still trying to understand. While the science is ongoing, there are worries about potential links to health issues like cancer, neurological symptoms, and disruptions in sleep patterns. Some people even experience electromagnetic hypersensitivity (EHS), causing skin rashes, tingling sensation, and difficulty concentrating. Given these concerns, it's crucial to take steps to minimize our exposure to EMFs and protect our well-being. While we can't completely avoid them in our modern world, there are practical ways to reduce our exposure:

- Limit your device usage and keep them away from your body when possible.
- Consider turning off Wi-Fi or switching to airplane mode, especially at night or during downtime which can minimize about ⅓ of exposure time.

- Designate EMF-free zones in your home, like bedrooms, by turning off electronics and unplugging appliances.
- Use wired connections like plug-in headphones over AirPods, ethernet cables, and corded phones instead of relying solely on wireless.
- Try setting up a Wi-Fi timer to help disconnect during certain times automatically.
- Practice safe habits like keeping cell phones away from your body during calls and using speakerphone or wired headsets.
- Explore shielding techniques with EMF-blocking, cases, fabrics, and paints to minimize exposure.
- Lastly, spend time outdoors in nature away from electronic devices to reduce overall EMF exposure.

By incorporating these habits into your daily routine, you can take proactive steps to minimize your exposure to EMFs and promote a healthier lifestyle.

Air Filters: Investing in Clean Air

Investing in an air filter is a fantastic way to ensure the air your family breathes is clean and healthy. Air filters remove contaminants like dust, mold spores, smoke, VOCs, allergens (such as pet dander and hair), bacteria, and even viruses. When choosing an air filter, look for one with a HEPA filter, and consider those with a VOC filter or PECO filter for added protection.

Additionally, using a vacuum cleaner fitted with a HEPA filter can help efficiently pick up small particles that get trapped in your home, further improving your indoor air quality. This combination of air filtration and effective vacuuming can create a healthier living environment for you and your loved ones.

Maintaining Ideal Humidity and Preventing Water Damage

Maintaining 35-50% humidity in your home is ideal for comfort and health. You can use a hygrometer to measure the humidity levels and ensure your air isn't too dry or too damp. If humidity levels stay high, it might indicate a leak, which can be detected using a whole-home leak detection device. These devices can help you monitor potential problem areas and prevent damage.

It's also wise to place water alarms in areas prone to flooding or leaks. Specifically, we recommend placing them near washing machines, water heaters, dishwashers, supply lines to automatic ice makers, and toilets. For example, place a sensor underneath or next to your washing machine to detect any cracked hoses or overflows during a cycle. Similarly, placing water sensors near water heaters, dishwashers, and toilets can alert you to leaks or overflows, helping you address issues before they cause significant damage. This proactive approach can save you from unexpected water damage and costly repairs.

Plants: Nature's Air Purifiers

Plants are not only beautiful to look at but also incredibly beneficial for our health. They improve air quality by eliminating pollutants and have even been known to boost mood and relieve stress. Some of the best indoor plants for cleaning the air include bamboo plants, English ivy, snake plants, spider plants, pothos, aloe vera, and peace lilies. Something to consider is that potted plants often mold, so mold-sensitive people do better with hydroponic setups, like clippings in water. Incorporating these plants into your home can create a healthier, more enjoyable living environment.

Lights and Their Impact on Well-being

Lighting plays a significant role in our daily lives and can greatly impact our well-being. Here are some important things to know about different types of lights and how they affect us:

LED lights are common in many households, but did you know that their rapid flicker can make us or our children feel overwhelmed and distracted? You can test this flicker by recording the light with your phone in slow-motion mode. If you see a rapid flicker, it might be affecting your comfort and concentration.

Incandescent lights are known for their warm and steady glow. Unfortunately, they're being phased out due to energy regulations. However, full-spectrum incandescent bulbs are still one of the best options because they don't flicker. Although they don't last as long as LEDs, they provide a more stable light that's easier on the eyes.

For a more calming and healthier lighting environment, consider using flicker-free or non-blue light bulbs. These types of bulbs can help reduce eye strain and create a more soothing atmosphere. These lights are longer lasting and easier to come by.

In your decorative lights, opt for incandescent or red bulbs. These create a warm, relaxing ambiance that's perfect for winding down in the evening.

Blue light exposure in the evening can interfere with your sleep. Try turning off all blue lights a few hours before bed. This can help your body produce melatonin, the hormone that regulates sleep.

Going back to basics with candlelight during dinner can create a cozy and calming atmosphere. It's a simple way to reduce blue light exposure and enjoy a more relaxing evening.

By being mindful of the types of lights you use in your home, you can create a more comfortable and health-friendly environment for you and your family.

Carpets, Pillows, Curtains, Furniture:

When it comes to carpets, pillows, curtains, and furniture, opting for natural materials can make a world of difference in minimizing toxins in your home. Look for items made from 100% cotton, jute, linen, or wool, as these are natural materials. For furniture, consider materials like solid wood, bamboo, rattan, reclaimed wood, metal, or glass.

But here's the cherry on top: look out for pieces with third-party certifications like Greenguard Gold, Oeko-Tex Standard 100, FSC,

GOTS, and GOLS. These certifications ensure that the products have been rigorously tested for harmful chemicals, giving you peace of mind.

When picking out household essentials, prioritize items that are free of formaldehyde and VOCs (volatile organic compounds), as these chemicals can be toxic. Whether it's paint, carpet, decor, or furniture, choosing toxin-free options can contribute to a healthier home environment.

2.2 Detoxifying Your Bedroom for Better Sleep

In your bedroom, consider adding elements of nature to your decor, like plants and natural fiber items, along with a HEPA air filter. These simple changes can create a peaceful and healthy sleep environment that supports restful sleep and overall well-being.

Creating a restful and toxin-free sleep environment is essential for overall health and well-being. Since we spend about a third of our lives sleeping, it's essential to ensure that our pillows, beds, and bedding are free from toxins, and dust mites. Start by investing in non-toxic pillows covers, pillows, sheets, mattress covers, and mattresses made from materials like organic cotton, sateen, linen, wool, tencel, lyocell, or latex.

Many traditional mattresses are treated with petroleum-based flame retardants and often contain synthetic materials that can off-gas over time and impact our health negatively. The concern with flame retardants is how they are made, using formaldehyde, polyurethane foams, glues, toxic perfumes, and other adhesives, which are harmful to our overall health and well-being. Exposure to flame retardant chemicals has been linked to serious health issues, including cancer, neurotoxicity, thyroid disease, and decreased fertility, as well as deficits in motor skills, attention, and IQ in children.

While mattresses are required to contain flame retardants for safety standards, it's important to choose options with natural and safe alternatives like latex, wool, and rayon.

When it comes to mattresses, it's important to know that they can be either organic, meaning non-toxic, or not. Even though CertiPUR like certifications indicate that the foams used are less toxic than regular ones, it is really not enough to ensure the off-gassing isn't going to harm us, our children, and our pets.

The best option would be to opt for a fully organic mattress. While it might take a little time to get used to the different feel and might require some extra comfort layering, these mattresses generally last much longer and are completely free of toxins.

If a fully organic mattress isn't an option right now, an organic barrier cover can be a great alternative to keep toxins from escaping. Mattresses and bedding made from natural materials can help create a healthier sleep environment for you and your family.

Candles and Synthetic Fragrances

To ensure a cleaner and safer environment, consider opting for candles made from beeswax. Additionally, choose essential oils that are pure and organic. Many scented candles contain synthetic fragrances and other toxins that can pollute the air in your home and your body. For home "fragrances" opt for herbal hydrosols. Your bedroom will feel both inviting and healthy with these simple swaps.

Natural Family Planning (NFP)

Also known as fertility awareness-based methods, offers a holistic and gentle approach to family planning that resonates with mindful living and environmental consciousness. By empowering individuals and couples to understand and work with their bodies' natural rhythms, NFP provides a safe, effective, and eco-friendly alternative to hormonal contraception and invasive fertility treatments.

These methods involve observing signs such as basal body temperature, cervical mucus, and menstrual cycle patterns to determine fertility status. The benefits of NFP: it's hormone-free, environmentally friendly, encourages a deeper understanding of the body's natural cycles and fertility signs, is cost-effective, and offers relationship and health benefits by avoiding hormonal contraceptives.

Fertility monitors, charting software, fertility awareness apps, and NFP programs offered are 93% effective with typical use and 98% with perfect use. Educational resources, classes, and online platforms are available to learn about different NFP methods and effectively track fertility signs which would be highly recommended. Embracing NFP methods allows individuals and couples to prioritize health, harmony, and mindfulness in their reproductive choices while minimizing their impact on the ecosystem. For more information on lubricants, prophylactics, and feminine care, refer to the bathroom section of this book.

2.3 The Kitchen Haul: Swapping for Safer Cookware, Utensils, and Cleaners

In the heart of our homes lies the kitchen, where we not only prepare meals but also nourish our bodies and connect with loved ones. The kitchen is a hotspot for toxins, from the cookware we use to the food we consume there are numerous opportunities to make healthier choices.

Let's start with cookware. Traditional non-stick pans may release harmful fumes when heated due to their coating of perfluorinated chemicals (PFCs). Safer alternatives are stainless steel, cast iron, or ceramic cookware.

In addition to cookware, it's essential to pay attention to other kitchen essentials such as food containers, dish soap, cooking tools, and even parchment paper. Look for products that are free from harmful chemicals and crafted from safe materials.

Favorite swaps to get you started:

- Non-stick pans → stainless steel, cast iron, or ceramic options.
- Plastic containers, cups → glass, and avoid heating food in plastic or styrofoam, wrap in cloth or beeswax reusable wraps. Mason jars are a favorite of mine.
- Microwave → heating food on the stove or in a 100% stainless steel toaster oven, or glass/100% stainless air fryer.
- Plastic utensils and tools → wood, stainless steel, or BPA-free silicone materials
- Name brand dish soap → without dyes or fragrances, biodegradable, biocompatible, concentrated all-purpose cleaner for multiple household tasks.
- Paper towels and napkins → reusable options like Swedish towels and cloth napkins.
- Aluminum foil→ Unbleached parchment paper.
- Produce cleaner -> concentrated all-purpose cleaner, Baking soda, lemon, and vinegar.
- Bleach -> Hypochlorous acid (HOCL) the disinfecting ingredient as effective as bleach, and the same substance your immune system produces to fight infections. Nonstriping and PH balanced (also great for acne, dermatitis, hand cleaner, and wounds).

Household Waste:

Managing household waste can be lessened with a little conscious repurchasing! Opt for products with less packaging, buy in bulk and you'll be amazed at how much trash you cut down. Plus, composting your kitchen scraps not only reduces waste but also gives you rich, nutrient-filled soil for your plants. And here's a tasty tip: save those vegetable peels and bones to make a hearty, nutritious bone broth—a delicious way to reduce waste and get more out of your groceries.

Simmer meat stock on low for 4-8 hours with salt. Add veggie scraps in the last hour and herbs in the last 30 minutes. Voila—you've got liquid gold! It's perfect for soups, stews, or just sipping to optimize the health of your gut microbiome.

Water Quality:
Finally, don't forget about the water you use for cooking and drinking. Invest in a reliable water filter to remove contaminants such as chlorine, heavy metals, fluoride, and pesticides. For drinking, the best resource is natural spring water, a Berkey filter and the third best is the reverse osmosis method then adding in minerals such as redmond or Celtic sea salt. Modern farming methods have depleted and stripped away essential trace minerals & other nutrients that are key to maintaining balance, good health, and vitality. These nutrients help restore electrolytes, relieve muscle cramps, support healthy joints, bones, energy, metabolic, mood support, and so much more. This is why now in modern society we need to add nutrients back into our drinking water for proper mineral absorption.

With these simple changes, we can transform our kitchen into a healthier, safer space for cooking and gathering.

2.4 Decoding Food: Having Healthier Eating Habits

In our journey toward healthier eating, it's easy to feel overwhelmed by the constant stream of dietary advice and a large variety of food industry options. Even when we're making small, positive changes, it can sometimes feel like those efforts aren't significant enough. BUT THEY ARE! One key message I want to emphasize is the importance of gradually developing habits around eating balanced meals most of the time. **A balanced meal includes a variety of nutrients: vegetables for fiber, protein, carbohydrates, and healthy fats.** One rule of thumb is to go for food that spoils quickly because that means it's real food, unprocessed, and most natural.

While there may be pressure to adhere to strict diet fads, I want to alleviate that pressure and encourage a more relaxed approach to eating. For example; If you are a daily soda drinker and cut your habit by half, celebrate that. If you buy a processed salad dressing but it's enticing you to eat vegetables, that makes a difference. Celebrate your wins. It's important to remember that small changes can lead to significant improvements in our health and well-being.

I will go into the hierarchy of what I believe can be feasible to all then go into detail as to what is the best option but all pressure aside ... **I believe focusing on eating real, unprocessed foods in each meal containing a protein, vegetable, carbohydrate, and fat is the most important when it comes to diet.** I then will go into how to choose the best form of those food types. I also want to reiterate that improving nutrition is only a piece to a healthy life where things like adequate sleep, drinking enough water, engaging in fitness, and managing stress are an all-encompassing way to a happy life. The key is consistency, not perfection, on the journey to a happier, healthier life.

Label Reading and Marketing Gimmicks

Knowing how to accurately read labels can make it easier to understand the ingredients in your food and make healthier choices, limiting chemical preservatives and additives. The largest food distributors prioritize profits, leading to confusion through misleading marketing tactics. Food is meant to be life-giving; fast, cheap, and convenient options are mostly not healthy. **Always look at the ingredient list. If you recognize and understand all the ingredients, it's likely a good choice.**

Don't be sold by the front of a package, always look at the ingredient list. If you can look at the ingredient list and know what everything is then this is a good pick. Greenwashing occurs when a company tries to trick consumers into thinking a packaged food is healthy. The front of the package may look appealing with nature scenes, green pastures, happy animals, and words like "natural," "healthy," and "fat-free," but there are no regulations governing these claims. Just because a label makes certain claims doesn't guarantee that the product is a healthy choice. Instead, **focus on the back of the package.**

Look out for preservatives, high fructose corn syrup, artificial dyes, seed oils or hydrogenated oils and artificial "natural" flavors, as they have no nutritional value and contribute to the diseases and systemic inflammation issues we are seeing with so many.

Opt for Healthier Alternatives:

Instead of canola, corn, sunflower, safflower, and soybean oils → olive or avocado oil, butter, or beef tallow

Instead of high fructose corn syrup, natural flavors, and refined white sugar → maple syrup, coconut sugar, honey, monk fruit, sugar cane or stevia.

Choose foods that perish quickly, as minimal processing and preservatives are indicators of healthier options. Our bodies thrive on natural, living, and whole (perishable) foods. Avoid products with a long shelf life, as they often contain additives our bodies don't need.

Produce (Vegetable, Fiber):

When shopping for produce, **the best place to start is the perimeter of the grocery store** where you'll find the freshest and most perishable items. Opt for foods that spoil quickly, as they are closer to their natural source, our earth. Are you catching my message yet?!

Cleaning your produce is a great way to help remove chemical residue and dirt: soaking 1:3 white vinegar or 1 teaspoon to every 2 cups of cold water for 5-10 mins. Using a large salad spinner or a large bowl with a cotton dish towel is my favorite way to dry. You can also use a non-toxic spray and then rinse for produce as well. Make sure to rinse in filtered water.

DIY Produce Cleaner is a great way to help remove chemical residue and dirt

- 1 part Vinegar
- 3 part water
- Soak 5-10 minutes
- Use a large salad spinner, large bowl, or flat cotton dish towel to dry
- (Alternatively, you can use a non-toxic spray and rinse method.)

Produce Budgeting

When budgeting, consider buying in bulk or opting for frozen organic produce, which is often more affordable and picked at peak season. Be mindful of the "Dirty Dozen," a list of produce items with the highest amounts of pesticides, which you should prioritize buying organic:

- Strawberries
- Blueberries
- Cherries
- Apples
- Nectarines
- Pears
- Peaches
- Grapes
- Spinach
- Kale/Collard Greens
- Bell and Hot Peppers
- Green Beans
- Potatoes

For optimal health, shop and eat locally. Farmers' markets are excellent places to find fresh, in-season foods. Here's a seasonal guide for California produce:

- Winter: Potatoes, beets, yams, turnips, carrots, kale, bok choy, onions, avocados, apples, kiwi, melons, mushrooms, celery, radishes, leafy greens, brussel sprouts, corn, cucumbers, crab, halibut, seabass, white fish, prawns, oysters.
- Spring: Onions, garlic, leafy greens & herbs, mushrooms, celery, cherries, oranges, apricots, strawberries, plums, melons, snap peas, broccoli, carrots, avocados, artichokes, cabbage, beets, asparagus, brussel sprouts, lobster, shrimp, crab, rockfish, albacore, tuna, seabass, swordfish.
- Summer: Tomatoes, eggplant, peppers, bell peppers, radishes, artichokes, corn, cucumbers, carrots, snap peas, potatoes, leafy greens, herbs, onions, garlic, ginger, watermelon, peaches, plums, strawberries, blueberries, mangoes, pineapples, almonds, walnuts, beans, crab, tuna, albacore, prawns, halibut, swordfish, salmon, shrimp, seabass.
- Autumn: Cauliflower, squash, zucchini, artichokes, bok choy, kale, potatoes, radishes, brussel sprouts, tomatoes, garlic, onions, ginger, leafy greens, herbs, papaya, grapes, beans, pomegranate, melons, pears, apples, tuna, albacore, halibut, shrimp, prawns, seabass.

Starting a home garden, no matter the size, can also be highly beneficial. Organic gardening uses natural composting methods instead of synthetic fertilizers and incorporates techniques like using beneficial insects, birds, crop rotation, traps, weeding, mulches, and crop rotation for weed management. If you can start a garden of any size at home that would also be advantageous.

Protein

When it comes to protein, it's important to purchase mindfully, focusing on quality over quantity. A little bit of high-quality, responsibly sourced meat can provide bioavailable nutrients, being more beneficial for your health and the planet.

Animal Protein

Quality Over Quantity: Meat raised on pastures by family farmers who use regenerative farming practices are nutrient-rich and regenerative to our land. Properly raised and rotated grass-fed cattle are necessary for maintaining a healthy ecosystem. Grass and pasture-raised organic livestock allow for regenerative agricultural practices and rotational grazing, which help to preserve nutrients in the land and animals.

Look for labels indicating 100% grass-fed and finished beef, pasture-raised chickens, and pork that feed on their natural diet of bugs and forage, offering more flavor and nutrients. Wild-caught seafood is also an excellent choice.

Local and Sustainable: If not available nearby search for local family farm delivery companies that prioritize animal welfare and land stewardship. Supporting these farms ensures that you're getting the best quality while contributing to sustainable agriculture.

Dairy Products: Opt for organic, grass-fed, hormone, and antibiotic-free dairy products. A2 cows or raw milk can be easily digested for some. Raw milk is a complete protein packed with enzymes, containing more nutrients and healthy bacteria; benefiting gut flora. The enzymes and healthy bacteria that are mostly broken down through pasteurization are beneficial to the gut flora helping those with lactose intolerance, autoimmunity, and allergies.

Eggs: Another excellent source of protein is pasture-raised eggs, which are more nutritious, flavorful, and the best choice.

Plant Protein

Plant-based proteins are also valuable and should not be overlooked. The highest sources of plant protein include:

- Beans (kidney, fava, lima, mung, soy, edamame)
- Chickpeas

- Lentils
- Tofu and tempeh
- Whey
- Broccoli, spinach, and Brussels sprouts

When buying beans, consider purchasing dry beans in bulk or stocking up on canned beans when they're on sale. These are cost-effective ways to ensure you always have a protein-rich option on hand.

By focusing on these high-quality, sustainable protein sources, you can improve your diet and overall health while supporting practices that are better for the environment.

Carbohydrates/Grains: Choosing Whole Foods

When it comes to carbohydrates and grains, choosing whole foods over processed options is always the best choice. If it grows from the ground, that is your best source. Buying in bulk is a fantastic way to get high-quality ingredients while keeping costs down. Think potatoes, squash, quinoa, barley, legumes, beans, and whole grains.

Wholesale options, like Costco, are excellent for purchasing organic starches and legumes at affordable prices. I love my bread maker—it's a quick and easy way to select high-grade ingredients and avoid preservatives. My favorite combination of grains includes Italian flour, einkorn flour, almond flour, and a 1:1 gluten-free flour blend.

For the best quality, and if it's financially feasible, consider sourcing from farmers who grow, harvest, and mill the grains in-house, family-owned. To mill wheat at home, you can use a high-powered blender, food processor, coffee grinder, or electric grain mill.

Healthy Fats

Healthy fats are essential for maintaining overall health and well-being. They play a key role in energy production, cell growth, hormone regulation, and nutrient absorption. Plus, they support brain and heart health and help control inflammation. Despite their benefits, fats have often been stigmatized due to their association with obesity and heart disease. However, understanding the differences between unhealthy and healthy fats can improve health outcomes.

Healthy fats, such as monounsaturated and polyunsaturated fats, are found in foods like avocados, nuts, seeds, olive oil, and fatty fish. These fats are beneficial and should be included in your diet. On the other hand, trans fats and excessive saturated fats, often found in processed foods, have been linked to negative health effects. Oils like canola, corn, sunflower, safflower, and soybean are highly processed and inflammatory. Instead, opt for healthier alternatives like olive oil, avocado oil, butter, and beef tallow.

Canola, corn oil, sunflower oil, safflower, soybean oil → olive and avocado oil is best, butter, beef tallow

Processed foods often contain unhealthy fats, so it's important to check the ingredients on the packaging. Moving past the stigma surrounding fats requires a shift in perspective and education. By emphasizing the positive impact of healthy fats in a balanced diet, you can make better choices for your health. Choose good fats and steer clear of processed fats for a healthier lifestyle.

Organic:

When it comes to our food, the laws surrounding the use of pesticides, antibiotics, hormones, and additives are surprisingly sparse. While shopping organic might seem like a luxury, it's worth considering the hidden costs impacting our health, our soil, and our farmers.

Conventional produce often contains fewer nutrients, supports mass production, and includes genetically modified crops that don't promote the regeneration of our ecosystem. By choosing organic whenever possible, you're not only nourishing your body but also supporting sustainable farming practices that benefit everyone.

When you eat organic you minimize your exposure to pesticides and chemicals. Organic farming reduces greenhouse gasses and decreases chemicals in the soil and water. By not spraying pesticides this helps our local ecosystems like birds, bees, and butterflies, which are essential to the health of our planet. Buying organic shows a demand for it and supports farmers who care about the conditions of our food, animals, and ultimately contributing to the longevity of our ecosystem and existence.

Core Food Message:
With the constant influx of diet fads, fear-mongering, and conflicting advice about what to eat, it's easy to feel overwhelmed. However, maintaining a healthy diet doesn't have to be complicated. The core message of a healthy diet is simple: **Focus on eating real food that isn't prepackaged or preserved. Aim to include a vegetable, protein, carbohydrates, and healthy fat in each meal. Organic or inorganic. The main message is getting in the 4 core food types for sustained health and energy.** By prioritizing whole foods you ensure you're getting the most nutritional value, free from the additives and preservatives found in processed foods.

Practical Steps to Implementing a Balanced, Whole-Food Diet

1. Balanced Meals for optimal health/Embracing real whole foods: vegetable, protein, carbohydrate, and healthy fat as primary foods on the plate.
2. Read Labels: When purchasing packaged items, choose those with the fewest ingredients and no artificial additives. This helps in minimizing the intake of unhealthy fats and preservatives.
3. Plan Ahead: Prepare meals at home using fresh ingredients. This not only ensures control over what goes into your food but also helps in maintaining a balanced intake of vegetables, proteins, carbs, and healthy fats.

3

Non-Toxic Cleaning & Laundry: A Healthier Choice for You and the Environment

Many conventional cleaning products contain a cocktail of toxic chemicals that can harm both our health and the environment. Fortunately, there are plenty of non-toxic alternatives available. Start by identifying the harmful ingredients in your current cleaning products and replacing them with safer options. Look for products that are free from ingredients such as phthalates, ammonia, chlorine, and synthetic fragrances.

Buying Concentrated Products: For affordability and practicality, consider buying concentrated cleaning products that can be used for multiple purposes. A gallon of non-toxic concentrated all-purpose cleaner can be watered down according to the target space and purpose, optimizing usage. You can enhance its effectiveness by adding natural ingredients like baking soda or vinegar for tougher stained areas.

I use this concentrate for mopping, laundry, dishes, cars, hand soap, and more. My favorite spray, which is stronger and safer than bleach, is hypochlorous acid (HOCL). HOCL is naturally produced in the human body to fight off viruses, bacteria, and fungi. This is my favorite go-to surface & bathroom cleaner (more on that in the first aid section).

Essential Cleaning Tools: Having the right cleaning tools is important. I recommend a stainless steel chainmail scrubber, scraping tools, silicone bottle scrubbers, bamboo dish scrubbers, Swedish dish towels, and a spin mop. You can also repurpose old towels and cloths as rags by cutting them to size for cleanup jobs.

Laundry Tips: For laundry, choose detergents that are free from harsh chemicals and synthetic fragrances. Consider switching to natural alternatives such as concentrated soaps as detergent, pre-wash spot cleaning with a toothbrush, and wool balls for the dryer, which are gentle on both your clothes and the environment. Air-drying clothes can reduce energy use and make clothes last longer. Retractable clotheslines are a great space-saving option.

<u>Laundry Detergent</u>

- 1 cup of washing soda (sodium carbonate)
- 1 cup of borax
- 1 bar of castile soap (or any mild soap), grated
- Optional: Essential oils for fragrance (e.g., lavender, lemon)

<u>DIY Stain Remover</u>

- 1 part hydrogen peroxide
- 1 part concentrate soap (e.g., Suds)
- 1 part baking soda

DIY Cleaning Products: You can make your non-toxic cleaning products using simple ingredients such as vinegar, baking soda, and essential oils. Not only are these homemade cleaners effective, but they're also more affordable and eco-friendly.

DIY Multipurpose Cleaning Spray

- 2 cups distilled water
- 1/4 cup white vinegar
- 1/4 cup rubbing alcohol (at least 70% concentration)
- 1 tablespoon baking soda
- 10-15 drops of essential oils (e.g., lemon, lavender, tea tree)

DIY Glass Cleaner

- 1 cup distilled water (or 1 cup vodka 2 cups water)
- ¼ cup white vinegar
- 1 tablespoon cornstarch (optional, for reducing streaking)
- 2 cups water
- 5-10 drops of essential oils (optional, for fragrance)

DIY Dusting Spray

- 1 cup distilled water
- 1/4 cup white vinegar
- 1 tablespoon olive oil (or any other vegetable oil)
- 5-10 drops of essential oils (optional, for fragrance)

Bathroom Cleaning Recipes:

Keeping your shower/bath space clean is very important, keeping dry around your shower items and in the corners is important in avoiding mold and grime. I would recommend using hypochlorous acid as a cleaner, Dr. Bronner Sal Suds soap, and/or a combination of these simple DIY recipes:

DIY Tile & Grout Cleaner

- 7 cup water
- ½ cup baking soda
- ⅓ cup lemon juice
- ¼ cup vinegar

DIY Shower Glass Cleaner

- Lemon (cut in half and use as a scrubber)
- Dip the lemon in Baking soda
- Use to apply to glass
- Leave for 30 minutes
- Scrub
- Rinse

DIY Bathroom Scrub

- ½ cup baking soda
- ½ cup Castile or concentrate
- 1 cup water

DIY Unclog & Deodorizer for Sink & Shower Drains

- 1 cup baking soda
- 2 cups vinegar
- Cover with cloth - 10 minutes
- Rinse with boiling water
- Add lemon juice to remove the odor

Creating your cleaning products can be a great way to save money, reduce waste, and minimize exposure to potentially harmful chemicals. Here's a basic list of ingredients commonly used in DIY cleaning products:

1. Baking Soda: A versatile cleaner and deodorizer that can be used for scrubbing surfaces, absorbing odors, and more.
2. White Vinegar: Effective for cutting through grease, removing stains, brightening whites, softening fabric, repelling pet hair, deodorizing and disinfecting surfaces.
3. Castile Soap: A gentle, plant-based soap that can be used as a base for many homemade cleaning solutions.
4. Hydrogen Peroxide: A natural disinfectant that can be used to kill bacteria and viruses. It's particularly useful for whitening surfaces.
5. Lemon Juice: Contains citric acid, which can help cut through grease and grime. It also adds a fresh scent to your cleaning solutions.
6. Olive Oil: Great for making homemade furniture polish or for conditioning wood surfaces.
7. Washing Soda (Sodium Carbonate): Similar to baking soda but stronger, washing soda is effective for cutting through tough grease and stains.
8. Citric Acid: Helps to remove hard water stains and soap scum. It's often used in homemade dishwasher detergents and toilet bowl cleaners.
9. Rubbing Alcohol: A disinfectant that can be used to kill bacteria on surfaces. It also helps to evaporate quickly, leaving surfaces streak-free.
10. Cornstarch: Can be used to make homemade carpet cleaners and as a natural alternative to talcum powder for absorbing odors.
11. Coconut Oil: Used in some homemade furniture polishes and wood conditioners.
12. Salt: Works as a gentle abrasive for scrubbing surfaces like sinks, pots, and pans. It's also effective for removing stains and odors.

13. Distilled Water: Often used as a base for homemade cleaning solutions to ensure purity and minimize mineral deposits on surfaces.
14. Vegetable Glycerin: Helps to stabilize and thicken homemade cleaning solutions. It can also add moisture to homemade hand soaps and lotions.
15. Witch Hazel: A natural astringent that can be used in homemade glass cleaners and surface disinfectants.
16. Vodka: Has disinfectant properties due to its high alcohol content. It can be used in homemade air fresheners and as a fabric refresher.
17. Borax: Acts as a natural cleaner, stain remover, and deodorizer. It's commonly used in laundry detergents and multipurpose cleaners.
18. Beeswax: Used in homemade furniture polish and wood conditioners to add shine and protection to wood surfaces.
19. Grapefruit Seed Extract: Contains antimicrobial properties and is often added to homemade cleaners for its ability to kill germs and bacteria.
20. Essential Oils: These add natural scent to your cleaning products and some, like tea tree oil, have antimicrobial properties. Popular options include lavender, lemon, tea tree, and eucalyptus oils.
21. Tea Tree Oil: Known for its antimicrobial properties, tea tree oil is often added to homemade cleaners to help kill germs and bacteria.
22. Rosemary Oil: Adds a pleasant fragrance to homemade cleaners and may also have antimicrobial properties.
23. Peppermint Oil: Provides a refreshing scent to homemade cleaners and can help deter pests like ants and spiders.

4

Nurturing Your Body: Understanding The Good, The Bad, and The Toxic

Our bodies come into contact with a multitude of toxins every day, from the personal care products we use to the materials we wear. In this chapter, we'll explore how to reduce our exposure to toxins in the bathroom and beyond.

4.1 Natural Skin, Hair, and Dental Care Solutions

Enhancing Water Quality and Care: If you're not getting natural spring water from your faucet, consider adding a shower head filter or a bath ball filter to your bath faucet. The water in your shower can be a major culprit behind various hair and skin issues such as hair loss, dryness, itchy scalp, eczema, acne, aging, and rashes. A simple filter attachment can remove chlorine, heavy metals, and other contaminants that strip the vitality from your hair and skin. This natural shift can significantly enhance the vibrancy of your skin and hair.

Shower Skin & Hair Care: For body care, use natural soap or a prebiotic cleanser. Opt for hair products that are all-natural, chemical-free, paraben-free, and free of sodium lauryl sulfate, which are drying, clogging, and skin irritants. Natural hair care lines have come a long way and are just as effective.

Shaving and Hair Removal: To reduce consumption, consider a reusable razor that lasts. Sugaring waxing, which uses just sugar, water, and lemon, is a great natural eco alternative. You can make it at home, buy sugar wax online, or visit a professional for service. For shaving, the "Flawless Legs" electric shaver is ideal for everyday body shaving, dermaplaning razor for the face, and a Swedish steel razor with blade replacements for intimate areas. Castile and Sal Suds soap are also recommended. Laser hair removal, while not entirely "natural," can be a semi-permanent solution that reduces long-term product consumption.

Toilet Paper and Feminine Care

When it comes to personal hygiene products, especially those for feminine care and toilet paper, it's best to choose options that are free from chlorine, bleach, dyes, and fragrances. Opt for products made from organic cotton or bamboo, which are gentler on both your body and the environment.

For underwear, 100% cotton and natural cotton products are ideal. For feminine care items, medical-grade silicone discs or cups are the safest and best options for reproductive health and the environment. Another eco-friendly and health-conscious choice would be period panties. However, it's essential to be mindful since some period panties can be made with plastics and harmful toxins. Look for a company that is B Corp certified or offers organic products. My personal favorites are an Australian company for the menstrual disc and a Canadian company for the undies. If you use pads or tampons, search for products that are chlorine and bleach-free. The toxins allowed in menstrual hygiene products are shocking, and switching to safer alternatives is imperative to your overall and reproductive health.

Additionally, consider adding a bidet to your hygiene routine. It's not only beneficial for the environment but also gentler on the skin (as long as it's not toxic water being used).

Lubricants

The reproductive area is one of the most sensitive parts of the body, with a high concentration of blood vessels and lymph for both men and women. Since this area is much more absorptive than other parts of the body the presence of chemicals and hormone-disrupting products is concerning and should be avoided.

Many lubricants have ingredients harmful to the reproductive system, especially to the female microbiome. Avoid fragrances, parabens, glycerin, and propylene glycol in lubricants, these can be skin irritants and kill healthy bacteria.

Safe alternatives include coconut oil, aloe vera gel, and vitamin E, but be mindful that reactions can vary; for instance, coconut oil's antimicrobial properties may not suit everyone. If any product feels aggravating, discontinue use immediately.

If it's safe to ingest it is most likely safe to use such as coconut oil, aloe vera gel, and vitamin E. It is important to note that just because an oil works for some it may not react the same to your body–for example, coconut oil is a very popular natural lubricant but it has antimicrobial properties which can be reactive to some.

Condoms

While the Natural Family Planning method is the most natural form, it's not feasible for everyone and not especially safe if you don't have a primary partner. Non-toxic condoms are made without harmful chemicals like parabens, glycerin, nonoxynol-9, benzocaine, lidocaine, and spermicides, which can irritate sensitive skin and disrupt hormonal balance. Condoms free from that are your ideal option. They are crafted from natural, eco-friendly materials like natural latex. These condoms provide a safer option for intimate moments, offering reliable protection without the risk of exposure to toxic substances. If something feels aggravating, always discontinue. Remember also, oil-based lubricants break down condoms so are not safe to use together, look for a water/silicon-based option.

Cranberry concentrate, D-Mannose, and fermented foods are also natural ways of improving the microbiome. Staying hydrated and eating healthy fats, especially omega 3 fatty acids, is also helpful. The female ovaries and male testes are major constituents of the Endocrine system, which we know regulates hormone production and function. This is a place I believe should be taken seriously with natural products. 100% Cotton underwear, natural cotton feminine care, and medical-grade silicone discs or cups are the best and safest forms for reproductive health.

Dental Care

There are hundreds of different bacteria in the mouth that make up your oral microbiome. They play a crucial role in our health. Immunity, digestion, and circulatory health (heart). Big-name brand oral care products often focus on killing bacteria using alcohol and fluoride. However, alcohol in toothpaste and mouthwash can be harsh on enamel and indiscriminately kills both good and bad bacteria.

Fluoride has been the gold standard for stronger, cavity-resistant teeth despite safety concerns. Flouride is an endocrine disruptor, and neurotoxin, affects the thyroid, is antimicrobial (killing good and bad bacteria), and impacts child brain development and IQ. A new non-toxic and biocompatible ingredient called hydroxyapatite is gaining popularity. Hydroxyapatite is a form of calcium that constitutes up to 97% of your tooth enamel and 70% of your bone and dentin. Recent studies have found hydroxyapatite to be as effective, if not more, than fluoride in reducing plaque and remineralizing enamel, particularly in children. Unlike fluoride, hydroxyapatite reaches the innermost part of the tooth, remineralizing enamel from within and effectively tackling plaque. Hydroxyapatite is beneficial for cavity prevention, enamel remineralization, tooth surface protection, restoring natural whiteness, and reducing dental hypersensitivity and pain.

4.2 Personal Care Essentials: Beauty Products: Skincare & Cosmetics

The bathroom is a huge area of the home where toxins abound, particularly in personal care products. Many conventional skincare, haircare, and cleaning products are packed with chemicals that can be harmful to your health. Did you know that the US bans only 30 ingredients, while Europe bans 1,300? It's estimated that 3,500 common ingredients could negatively impact our long-term health!

In the US, the skincare and body essentials industry is under-regulated. The FDA, which oversees cosmetics and skincare, has limited power to ensure product safety and sustainability. On average, women are exposed to 168 toxins daily in personal care products. That's why it's up to us to research the products we use daily. Here are some handy websites to check ingredient safety and learn more about what's in your products:

- INCIdecoder
- Paula's Choice Ingredient Checker
- Cosmetics Info

These sites are great starting points for checking your soon-to-be swaps. It can seem overwhelming at first, so I recommend doing ingredient checks as your current products run out or when you're ready to buy new ones. This approach keeps things manageable and helps you avoid the stress of tossing everything out at once.

Here are a few tips to make the transition smoother:

1. Read Labels: Start by examining the labels of your personal care

products. Opt for natural alternatives whenever possible.
2. <u>Avoid Harmful Ingredients</u>: Look for products free from parabens, phthalates, sulfates, and synthetic fragrances.
3. <u>Seek High-Quality Brands</u>: I highly recommend Credo Beauty for makeup. They ban over 3,000 ingredients based on safety and sustainability concerns.
4. <u>Join Communities</u>: Non-toxic Facebook groups and subreddits are excellent resources. You can get recommendations for safer alternatives to products you will love.

Remember, your skin is the largest organ in your body. What you apply to it has a direct impact on your internal health. That's why beauty care products are a top priority for swapping, as they are used daily and are highly absorbent.

Switching to cleaner products might mean letting go of some longtime favorites, but don't worry! Forums and review sites are your friends. Read reviews in detail to find products that meet your needs. Reach out to community pages for suggestions on non-toxic alternatives that have the qualities you love.

Stay positive! Making your few-ingredient essentials or buying in bulk is a great way to start. Not only are these DIY recipes effective, but they're also customizable and budget-friendly.

4.3 Homemade Beauty: Simple Recipes for Skincare

<u>Rosewater Facial Toner</u>: Mix distilled water with rose petals and simmer on low heat for about 30 minutes. Let it cool, strain out the rose petals, and pour the rose-infused water into a spray bottle. Use it as a hydrating and refreshing facial toner.

<u>Coconut Oil Makeup Remover</u>: Simply apply a small amount of coconut oil to a cotton pad and gently wipe away makeup. It's effective

and gentle on the skin you can also use jojoba, olive, or avocado oil). If it is too oily for you, you can do equal parts oil and witch hazel in a spray bottle.

Clay Face Mask: Mix clay powder (such as bentonite or kaolin) with water or apple cider vinegar until it forms a smooth paste. Apply it to your face and let it dry before rinsing off. Clay masks help draw out impurities and can leave your skin feeling fresh and clean.

Aloe Vera Gel Soothing Gel: Extract the gel from an aloe vera leaf and apply it directly to sunburns or irritated skin for soothing relief. Aloe vera has anti-inflammatory properties and can help heal damaged skin.

Olive Oil Nail and Cuticle Treatment: Massage olive oil into your nails and cuticles to moisturize and strengthen them. Olive oil is rich in vitamins and antioxidants, promoting healthy nail growth.

Castor Oil and Rosemary Hair Oil: 2 part castor oil 1 part rosemary-infused oil (or 5-6 drops of rosemary essential oil) If you're using rosemary-infused oil, you can make it by steeping dried rosemary leaves in a carrier oil like olive oil or coconut oil for a few weeks. Strain out the rosemary leaves before using the infused oil in your hair oil blend. If you're using rosemary essential oil, simply add 5-6 drops to the castor oil.

Lavender and Magnesium Flakes/ Epsom Salt Bath Soak: Combine magnesium Epsom salt with dried lavender buds and or a few drops of lavender essential oil for a relaxing bath soak. Epsom salt helps to relax muscles and reduce tension, while lavender promotes relaxation and calmness.

Peppermint and Tea Tree Oil Acne Spot Treatment: Mix a drop of tea tree oil with a drop of peppermint oil and apply it directly to blemishes as a spot treatment. Both oils have antimicrobial properties that can help reduce acne-causing bacteria to the skin.

Shea Butter Body Lotion: Melt shea butter in a double boiler, then mix in a carrier oil like jojoba or almond oil. Let it cool and solidify before whipping it into a creamy lotion. Shea butter is deeply moisturizing and great for dry skin.

Sugar Lip Scrub: Mix together sugar and coconut oil to create a gentle lip scrub. Rub it onto your lips in circular motions to exfoliate and moisturize.

These DIY beauty products are not only non-toxic but also cost-effective and customizable to suit your skin and hair needs. Always perform a patch test before using any new products, especially if you have sensitive skin.

4.4 Good Clothing Habits & Upcycling Clothing

Adopting good clothing habits can significantly reduce our exposure to harmful chemicals and minimize waste. Here are some practical tips to keep in mind:

Choose Natural Fibers: Opt for clothing made from natural fibers like cotton, linen, wool, and silk. These materials are generally free from harmful chemicals found in synthetic fabrics.

Read Labels: Check the labels for information on fabric content and care instructions. Avoid garments that require dry cleaning, as the chemicals used can be harmful to both you and the environment.

Wash Wisely: Use gentle, non-toxic detergents and avoid fabric softeners. Air-drying and washing your clothes in cold water and when possible can also extend their lifespan and reduce energy consumption.

Buy Secondhand: Thrift stores, consignment shops, and online marketplaces (thredUP, Nuuly) offer a treasure trove of pre-loved clothing. Buying secondhand reduces demand for new clothing production and helps keep perfectly good items out of landfills.

Clothing Swaps: Organize or participate in clothing swaps with friends, family, or your community. It's a great way to refresh your wardrobe without spending money or contributing to waste. Plus, it's a fun social activity that promotes sharing and sustainability.

Mindful Shopping: When you do need to buy new clothes, invest in high-quality, timeless pieces that you'll love and wear for years. Look for brands committed to sustainable and ethical practices.

Upcycling Clothing

Upcycling is all about creativity and resourcefulness, giving old clothes new life instead of discarding them. Transform old t-shirts into tote bags, jeans into shorts, or fabric scraps into patchwork quilts. Use natural dyes to refresh faded garments or add unique designs with fabric paint. Simple alterations like sewing on new buttons, patching holes, or adjusting hems can also significantly extend the life of your clothing. Many of my old clothes become cleaning cloths for around the house or clothing I use for messy jobs. These fun and practical projects are satisfying and help cut down.

By upcycling your clothing, you can reduce waste, save money, and express your creativity. It's all about making small, thoughtful choices that add up to a big impact.

4.5 Natural First Aid and Holistic Remedies

Stocking a natural first aid kit with essential oils, herbal remedies, and other natural treatments is an excellent way to prepare for minor injuries and ailments. Essential oils such as lavender, tea tree, and peppermint have powerful healing properties and can be used to treat everything from cuts and scrapes to headaches and insect bites.

Hypochlorous acid spray is a safe, natural, non-toxic, and gentle molecule used in hospitals and hospitals worldwide to repair cuts, skin irritants, burns, and rashes.

Medicine Cabinet Essentials :

1. Calendula Cream or Salve: For cuts, scrapes, and minor skin irritations.
2. Activated Charcoal: For treating poisonings and digestive issues like gas and bloating.
3. Honey: For wound healing, burns, and soothing sore throats. Manuka honey is especially prized for its antibacterial properties.
4. Ginger: For nausea and upset stomach. You can include ginger candies or ginger tea bags.
5. Magnesium Flakes or Epsom Salt: For soaking sore muscles and relieving minor sprains and bruises.
6. Witch Hazel: For soothing insect bites, minor burns, and skin irritation.
7. Chamomile: For calming upset stomachs, promoting relaxation, and soothing skin irritations.
8. Dragon's Blood: Anti-inflammatory, antimicrobial, and wound-healing properties, making it a valuable addition to holistic first aid practices. It relieves pain and stops bleeding.
9. Bentonite Clay: detoxifying making it an effective remedy for drawing out fluid and infection from wounds while promoting circulation and healing. It can be used in a bath or a mask to reduce swelling and soothe inflammation.
10. Adhesive Bandages: bamboo or plant-based materials for covering small cuts and scrapes. Dragon's Blood or poltice from bentonite clay is a good bandage alternative. Be watchful of PFAs in conventional brands.
11. Gauze Pads, Tape, wound closure stickers: For larger wounds that need to be covered or sealed. Dragon's Blood or poltice from bentonite clay is good for sealing bigger wounds as well.
12. Cold & Heat Packs: For reducing swelling and relieving pain from

sprains and bruises. Heat to aid healing and warm circulation.
13. Hydrogen Peroxide: For cleaning wounds before applying first aid
14. Tea Tree Oil: An antiseptic for cuts, insect bites, and minor skin infections.
15. Lavender Essential Oil: For calming and soothing minor burns, insect bites, and headaches.
16. Eucalyptus Essential Oil: For relieving congestion and promoting easier breathing during colds and sinus infections.
17. Peppermint Essential Oil: For relieving headaches, nausea, and muscle tension. It can also be applied topically for cooling relief.

SUMMER DIY TRIO:

DIY Sunscreen

1 cup of lotion or body butter (you can use oils such as raspberry seed, carrot seed, macadamia, avocado oil, or olive oil that already have natural SPF in this 1 cup ration) melt then with a mask add zinc oxide to the lotion/butter based on your desired SPF level, stir to avoid clumping and store in room temperature or refrigeration (6-month shelf life)

Using 9 oz lotion with...	SPF 2-5	SPF 6-11	SPF 12-19	SPF >20
Nano-Zinc Oxide	.27oz =3%	.68oz=7.5%	1.08oz= 12%	1.8oz=20%
Non-Nano Zinc Oxide	.45oz= 5%	.9oz=10%	1.35oz= 15%	2.25oz=25%

Adapted from: Carly from Modern Hippie Inc.

DIY Bug Repellant:

- 10 drops of each citronella, eucalyptus, geranium, and lemongrass

essential oils (+- cedarwood, peppermint, rosemary, clove leaf, neem)
- 2 tablespoons witch hazel (or vodka as an alternative)
- 2 tablespoons of a carrier oil (such as coconut oil or jojoba oil)
- ½ cup distilled water
- vegetable glycerin 1 tsp. - preferred amount (optional, helps the oils mix better and moisturizes skin)
- Small spray bottle (preferably dark glass to protect the oils from light)

Reduce Chlorine Exposure:

- Coconut oil on the skin to protect the skin barrier before swim
- Vitamin C Spray: water and food-grade Vitamin C powder in a spray bottle to neutralize chlorine. Are able to also take internally.
- Rinse with Epsom Salt or Apple Cider Vinegar

5

Prioritizing Wellness

As we wrap up this pocketbook, it's essential to prioritize practices that support overall health and wellness. While minimizing our exposure to toxins is crucial; embracing holistic therapies and facilitating your body's natural shifts can enhance our well-being even further.

Our bodies are incredibly resilient and equipped with mechanisms to protect us. By optimizing these mechanisms, we can better withstand the inevitable exposures we encounter. Finding a balance that works for you is key. You can absolutely do things to help manage or prevent disease to lead to a higher quality of life. Sometimes, other interventions might be necessary, but these practices can significantly support your overall wellness.

It's essential to highlight practices that support overall health and wellness, alongside minimizing toxin exposure. In this chapter, we'll explore various holistic therapies and practices that can enhance your well-being.

5.1 Free Natural Shifts

Morning Light

Exposing your eyes to outdoor light as soon as you wake up is an easy and free way to synchronize your body. It might sound a bit "woo woo," but the benefits are substantial. Absorbing natural light upon waking helps regulate your body's internal clock (circadian rhythm), influencing sleep-wake cycles, hormones, cognition, stress response, and mood. It doesn't have to be sunny for it to be effective. You can enjoy your morning tea while doing it, and it doesn't need to be lengthy.

Nighttime Dark

At night, removing blue light exposure from electronic devices like smartphones and computers is crucial. Blue light can suppress melatonin production, essential for regulating sleep-wake cycles. Reducing blue light exposure before bedtime, through screen filters or avoiding electronic devices, allows your body to increase melatonin levels naturally, promoting better sleep quality. Consider setting your screen to red light mode and wearing blue-blocking lenses at night.

Sunlight or Red Light Therapy

Exposure to natural sunlight is essential for overall health, regulating circadian rhythms, boosting vitamin D levels, enhancing immune function, decreasing pain, decreasing stress perception, and reducing inflammation. A simple practice is to expose your eyes to outdoor light first thing in the morning.

Red light therapy, involving low levels of red or near-infrared light, offers benefits such as reduced inflammation, improved circulation, and enhanced wound healing.

Grounding/Nature

Grounding, or connecting with the Earth's surface, is a free reservoir of limitless healing. Research shows it mitigates inflammation, supports wound healing, enhances sleep, relieves pain, decreases inappropriate immune reactivity, and shifts your body out of fight-or-flight mode. Spending time in nature, whether in a park, forest, or beach, provides these benefits. Simply spending time barefoot on natural surfaces like grass, sand, or soil balances the body's electrical charge

Community & Human Connection

Human connection is a vital component of health that is often underestimated. Being part of a community and maintaining strong social ties can significantly impact your mental and physical well-being. Engaging with others provides emotional support, reduces feelings of loneliness, and increases your sense of belonging and purpose. Activities such as group exercises, community volunteering, or simply spending time with loved ones can create meaningful interactions that promote overall health.

By integrating these free and natural shifts into your lifestyle, you can enhance your well-being in profound ways.

5.2 Dr. Ashley's Personal Favorites

Acupuncture & Chinese Medicine

Acupuncture is an ancient Eastern medical therapy that involves the use of tiny sterile needles to activate key areas of the body to alleviate discomforts and optimize the health of body systems. Acupuncture is used to regulate the central nervous system, promote circulation, decrease inflammation, and lessen tension (including physical and emotional). Acupuncture treats pain by activating your brain to release your own body's natural painkillers (natural opioids), dump your body's natural feel-good hormones (serotonin and dopamine), and activate your parasympathetic nervous system (also known as "rest and digest") to enhance circulation throughout the body. With this holistic and balancing approach, the body can be highly receptive to healing.

I am a Doctor of Chinese Medicine and Acupuncture so I support this ancient modality through and through. I believe anyone can benefit from acupuncture, and I mean it! If you have any discomforts in the body acupuncture can help. Everything from inflammation, nervous system dysregulation, stress, pain, immunity dysfunctions, reproductive issues, mood shifts, digestion discomforts, life transitions, and even cosmetic aging are able to be addressed through acupuncture, the most integrative medicine. Acupuncture is an all-natural solution for instant relief and helps rebalance, recharge, and recover.

Rebounding

Rebounding, or jumping on a mini-trampoline, is a fun, low-impact exercise that promotes lymphatic drainage, helping flush out toxins, bacteria, dead cells, and other waste products. It improves balance, coordination, and motor skills which is great for our modern sedentary lifestyle. Rebounding also supports bone density, strength, and formation; supports cardiovascular health, and releases feel-good hormones like serotonin and dopamine, boosting your mood.

Castor Oil Packs

Castor oil packs are a holistic remedy involving a cloth soaked in castor oil applied to the skin. This practice helps enhance circulation, promote healing, improve lymphatic circulation, support detoxification, reduce inflammation, and provide pain relief. Many people use them to aid digestion and alleviate menstrual cramps. Applying castor oil packs on the liver is a gentle way to detoxify and stimulate the lymphatic system.

Sauna Therapy

Saunas have been used for centuries to promote detoxification and relaxation. Regular sauna sessions help eliminate toxins through sweat, improve circulation, enhance skin health, and boost immune function. A steam sauna deeply cleanses and hydrates the skin, helping to open pores, remove impurities, and promote a healthy, glowing complexion. Infrared saunas, which use infrared light to heat the body directly, are particularly effective for detoxification and are gentler on the body than traditional saunas.

Annual Parasite Cleanse

This is a realm I won't go into detail about here but we ALL have them. They are part of us and our ecosystem. I believe it is beneficial to periodically assist in flushing out the bad guys to help promote long-term gut health. Herbal remedies like wormwood, black walnut, clove, and papaya seeds are commonly used for their anti-parasitic properties. The cleansing process typically involves taking these herbs over one to three weeks, accompanied by a high-fiber diet and reduced sugar intake to enhance effectiveness. Supporting detoxification with hydration, regular bowel movements, probiotics, sauna therapy, and castor oil packs can further aid the cleanse. While beneficial for all, those pregnant, breastfeeding, or with chronic conditions should consult a healthcare provider before starting a cleanse to ensure safety and efficacy.

Colon hydrotherapy and coffee enemas assist in detoxifying the body, improve digestive health, and enhance overall well-being through the removal of toxins and the stimulation of the liver. This can be extremely beneficial for people who run on the constipation side. Going 2-3 times daily is optimal, and is especially important during a cleanse.

By focusing on these core elements, you can build a robust foundation for a healthier, more fulfilling life. I believe having consistency with these practices sets the foundation for a healthy life.

Basics of health & doing so with consistency

- Adequate Sleep
- Improve nutrition by eating balanced meals (Protein, Carbs, fat, vegetables)
- Drinking enough water

- Engaging in movement & fitness
- Stress management

6

Conclusion

Transitioning to a non-toxic lifestyle is not always easy, but the benefits far outweigh the challenges. By making conscious choices about the products we use, the materials we surround ourselves with, and the practices we prioritize, we can significantly reduce our exposure to toxins and improve our overall health and well-being. Whether it's switching to non-toxic cleaning products, choosing natural skincare, or exploring holistic therapies, every small step towards a toxin-free lifestyle brings us closer to optimal health and vitality. Here is also a quick reminder to use my QR code, which will send you to my vetted sources for each topic we spoke about along this journey in different facets of life.

Again…Thank you for joining me on this journey. Remember, the path to well-being doesn't have to be complicated or expensive. Sometimes, the simplest practices are the most effective. If this is something you enjoyed please share with a loved one. I'd be very appreciative if you left a favorable review for the book on Amazon too. Here's to your health and happiness!

CONCLUSION

References

Amaechi, B. T., AbdulAzees, P. A., Okoye, L. O., Meyer, F., & Enax, J. (2020). Comparison of hydroxyapatite and fluoride oral care gels for remineralization of initial caries: a pH-cycling study. *BDJ Open, 6*(1). https://doi.org/10.1038/s41405-020-0037-5

Aquarium of The Pacific & Seafood for the Future. (2014, March 12). *Seafood seasonality Southern California.* www.aquariumofpacific.org. https://www.aquariumofpacific.org/images/seafoodfuture/Seasonality_Southwest_KT_2014_03_12.pdf

Beautypedia Skin Care Ingredient Checker | Paula's Choice. (n.d.). Paula's Choice Skincare. https://paulaschoice.com/beautypedia-ingredient-checker

Butera, A., Gallo, S., Pascadopoli, M., Montasser, M. A., Latief, M. H. a. E., Modica, G. G., & Scribante, A. (n.d.). Home Oral Care with Biomimetic Hydroxyapatite vs. Conventional Fluoridated Toothpaste for the Remineralization and Desensitizing of White Spot Lesions: Randomized Clinical Trial. *International Journal of Environmental Research and Public Health/International Journal of Environmental Research and Public Health, 19*(14), 8676. https://doi.org/10.3390/ijerph19148676

Chemical Health Hazards | Public Health Ontario. (n.d.). Public Health Ontario. https://www.publichealthontario.ca/en/health-topics/environmental-occupational-health/health-hazards/chemical#:~:text=Health%20effects%20can%20range%20from,monitoring%20and%20address

REFERENCES

ing%20chemical%20hazards.

Collins, H. N., Johnson, P. I., Calderon, N. M., Clark, P. Y., Gillis, A. D., Le, A. M., Nguyen, D., Nguyen, C., Fu, L., O'Dwyer, T., & Harley, K. G. (2021). Differences in personal care product use by race/ethnicity among women in California: implications for chemical exposures. *Journal of Exposure Science & Environmental Epidemiology/Journal of Exposure Science and Environmental Epidemiology, 33*(2), 292–300. https://doi.org/10.1038/s41370-021-00404-7

Cosmetics Info. (2023, November 29). *Cosmetics info.* https://www.cosmeticsinfo.org/

Fats. (2023, October 27). www.heart.org. https://www.heart.org/en/healthy-living/healthy-eating/eat-smart/fats

Healthful habits. (n.d.). https://www.eatright.org/food/nutrition/healthy-eating

Healthy eating plate. (2024, May 9). The Nutrition Source. https://www.hsph.harvard.edu/nutritionsource/healthy-eating-plate/

How to make mineral sunscreen with zinc oxide — Modern Hippie Inc. (2024, January 27). Modern Hippie Inc. https://www.modernhippiehw.com/blog/homemade-moisturizing-sunblock-with-zinc-oxide

Human health issues related to pesticides | US EPA. (2023, October 4). US EPA. https://www.epa.gov/pesticide-science-and-assessing-pesticide-risks/human-health-issues-related-pesticides#:~:text=Some%2C%20such%20as%20the%20organophosphates,endocrine%20system%20in%20the%20body.

INCIDecoder - Decode your skincare ingredients. (n.d.). INCIDecoder. https://incidecoder.com/

Marcos, J. (2024, March 14). *Is hydroxyapatite better than fluoride? a dentist explains.* Biöm. https://betterbiom.com/blogs/learn/is-hydroxyapatite-better-than-fluoride

NCI Dictionary of Cancer Terms. (n.d.-a). Cancer.gov. https://www.cancer.gov/publications/dictionaries/cancer-terms/def/environmental-exposure

NCI Dictionary of Cancer Terms. (n.d.-b). Cancer.gov. https://www.cancer.gov/publications/dictionaries/cancer-terms/def/environmental-exposure

Oschman, J. L., Chevalier, G., & Brown, R. (n.d.). The effects of grounding (earthing) on inflammation, the immune response, wound healing, and prevention and treatment of chronic inflammatory and autoimmune diseases. *Journal of Inflammation Research*, 83. https://doi.org/10.2147/jir.s69656

Paszynska, E., Pawinska, M., Gawriolek, M., Kaminska, I., Otulakowska-Skrzynska, J., Marczuk-Kolada, G., Rzatowski, S., Sokolowska, K., Olszewska, A., Schlagenhauf, U., May, T. W., Amaechi, B. T., & Luczaj-Cepowicz, E. (2021). Impact of a toothpaste with microcrystalline hydroxyapatite on the occurrence of early childhood caries: a 1-year randomized clinical trial. *Scientific Reports, 11*(1). https://doi.org/10.1038/s41598-021-81112-y

Potential health effects of PFAS chemicals | ATSDR. (n.d.-a). https://www.atsdr.cdc.gov/pfas/health-effects/index.html

Potential health effects of PFAS chemicals | ATSDR. (n.d.-b). https://www.atsdr.cdc.gov/pfas/health-effects/index.html

Randall, P., & Randall, P. (2024, February 21). *Why ConcenTrace® Trace Mineral Drops is our best selling product.* Trace Minerals. https://www.traceminerals.com/blogs/post/why-concentrace%C2%AE-trace-mineral-drops-is-our-best-selling-product

Schrock, R. (2023, May 5). *Raw Milk and Why it is so Important — Vintage Meadows.* Vintage Meadows. https://www.vintagemeadows.farm/blog/2023/5/raw-dairy-and-why-it-is-so-important

Scripps Health. (2024, January 15). Cracking the produce sticker code. *Scripps Health.* https://www.scripps.org/news_items/4472-cracking-the-produce-sticker-code#:~:text=Organically%20grown%20fruits%20and%20vegetables,of%20the%20internationally%20standardized

REFERENCES

%20system.

Spanne, A. (2022a, December 2). What are PFAS? *EHN*. https://www.ehn.org/what-are-pfas-2656619391.html?gad_source=1&gclid=Cj0KCQjw8pKxBhD_ARIsAPrG45mrreafC8umnoUx639MJnLafhmPFRnh8At9OAWnRWQf0rE9PRYz2FkaAuXDEALw_wcB

Spanne, A. (2022b, December 2). What are PFAS? *EHN*. https://www.ehn.org/what-are-pfas-2656619391.html?gad_source=1&gclid=Cj0KCQjw8pKxBhD_ARIsAPrG45mrreafC8umnoUx639MJnLafhmPFRnh8At9OAWnRWQf0rE9PRYz2FkaAuXDEALw_wcB

Study: Replacing furniture and foam Reduces levels of toxic flame Retardants. (2021, March 24). Environmental Working Group. https://www.ewg.org/news-insights/news-release/2021/03/study-replacing-furniture-and-foam-reduces-levels-toxic-flame

What are Parabens and Phthalates?| VIDA Integrative Medicine. (n.d.). VIDA Integrative Medicine. https://carolyngeorgemd.com/blog/parabens-phthalates/#:~:text=Paraben%20%E2%80%93%20any%20of%20a%20group,products%2C%20yet%20here%20we%20are.

Why are there harmful chemicals in traditional mattresses? · Houston Natural Mattress. (2018, July 10). Houston Natural Mattress - Houston. https://www.houstonnaturalmattress.com/why-are-there-harmful-chemicals-in-traditional-mattresses/#:~:text=The%20main%20issue%20with%20traditional,%2C%20glues%2C%20and%20other%20adhesives.

World Health Organization: WHO. (2020, April 29). *Healthy diet*. https://www.who.int/news-room/fact-sheets/detail/healthy-diet

Printed in Great Britain
by Amazon